Surrendering to Rainbows

The Art and Science of Quieting the Noise of Chronic Pain

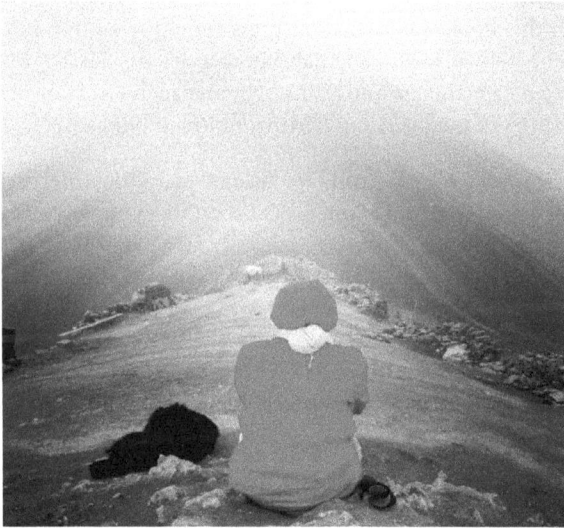

SABRINA CROUCH, PSY.D

ISBN: 978-1-64184-501-4 (Hardback)
ISBN: 978-1-64184-502-1 (Paperback)

Join My FACEBOOK Community!

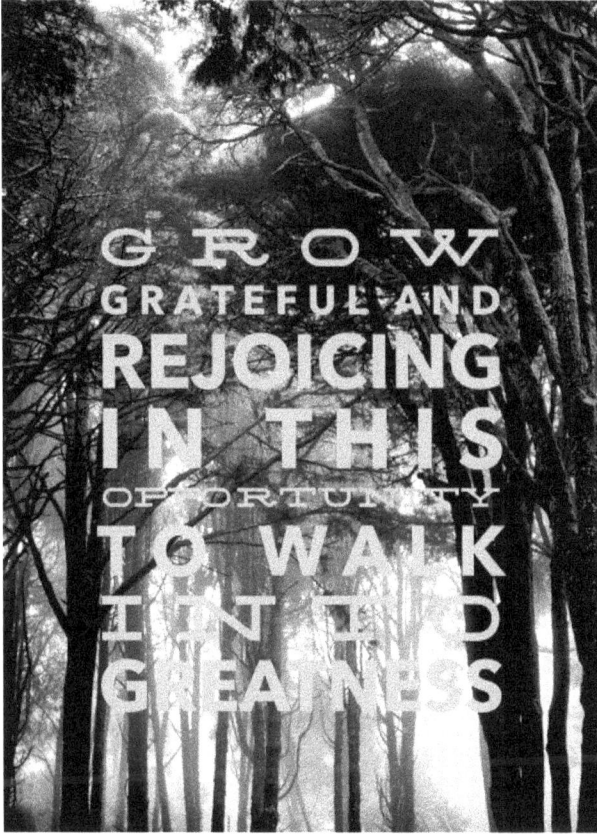

To get the best experience with this book, I encourage you to join my community. I have found that when readers who are on a similar journey are able to support each other through the process, they can implement changes faster and take the next steps needed to raise their consciousness and move forward with a renewed sense of courage and power.

Join my Facebook group GROW into Greatness:
facebook.com/groups/403532984162883

Table of Contents

Dedication

To those who have paved the way for me,
and those who walk beside me
as we learn to surrender to rainbows.

"Darling, I'm here for you.

Darling, I know you are there for me...and I'm so happy you are truly there.

Darling, I know you suffer...that is why I am here for you.

Darling, I suffer. I am trying my best to practice. Please help me."

Thich Nhat Hanh
Four Mantras of Relationship Success

Introduction

This book is a testament to my journey inward to manage chronic pain by learning to meditate. When I started this journey, it was all about me finding relief, but as my journey unfolded, I gained unexpected clarity. I believe it only takes one person to take a chance and have a breakthrough for others to see possibility. I hope I can be that person for you.

Surrendering to Rainbows is about abandoning everything we know about ourselves. Surrendering is not about giving up but letting go of patterns that no longer serve you. It's about what you do when your back is against the wall, you don't have a strategy, you don't know what else to do, and you think you are all out of options. It is about digging deep and being able to lift that emotional weight that has been holding you down. Once you do this, you will uncover unexpected blessings.

When I was first diagnosed with cervical stenosis, I feared being in a situation where I would feel powerless, restricted, or unable to take care of myself. I feared being dependent on others, and who takes care of the caretaker? Although the doctors stated it was mild, I couldn't imagine it being any worse. Stenosis left me with neck pain. There were days that my head felt so heavy that it was hard to stand up. The nerve sensations down my arm felt like shock waves that ended in my fingers. It left me with a hypersensitivity to touch (brushing up against a towel felt like I cut myself with a knife), sensitivities to temperature (if it was chilly outside, my left hand was ice cold, and if it was warm, it swelled), and what was worse for me was the unpredictable lack of movement. I would wake up, and my fingers would not move. I would stare at them, but it was like the signal from my brain was not going to my left hand. If I forced my fingers to move, it felt like I was breaking them, and I was in excruciating pain. This was on and off all day, every day. In the moments I was pain-free, I didn't know how to stay that way. Small tasks became a big deal. This condition left me frustrated, but despite this, I found a way. This pain gave me a new sense of purpose and a fire. I can now say this condition <u>could not</u> have happened to a better person. This book is about what I was willing to do to change aspects of my condition and what I discovered along the way. A journey is never predictable, and no two journeys are alike. Yes, I had setbacks, but the success and possibilities outweighed them every time. This book is an invitation for you to embark on a journey of your own. If you are willing to put aside convention, invest in the process, and see possibility, then this book is for you.

Like most people who think of incorporating meditation practices into their daily routine, I thought:

- *I can't sit still. There is no way I can meditate.*

- *I don't have time. If I don't put my time into other people, I will appear selfish and disappoint them.*

- *Does it work?*

- *Does it go against my religious practices?*

- *I'm always going to have "this condition," so why bother?*

Unfortunately, this is the mentality that would ensure that meditation wouldn't work. The first thing I want you to do is stop "trying" to meditate. For me, trying led to evaluating my progress, judging myself, and comparing my progress to others. If you focus on "doing meditation," it's like focusing on the end result instead of the small steps that are required to get there. Believe me, if you focus on the steps of the process, before you know it, you will be in the flow and meditating without realizing it. The first rule of meditating is to focus on being and not doing. In the beginning, I wasn't aware of this, but I discovered it along the way. I started this practice as a way to take my mind off the pain, but what I discovered was more profound. It not only improved my relationship with myself but also translated to my relationships with others and changed the lens I see the world through. In *Surrendering to Rainbows,* I outline the steps I took in preparing my mind, body, and spirit to embrace meditation. I found it through a formula I call the C's: Connection + Clarity x Compassion = Courage.

Part I: Connection explores knowledge of oneself and the importance of learning to recalibrate and self-regulate, which includes stillness, focused breathing, and heart/brain coherence.

Part II: Clarity explores the power of our thoughts, how we get locked into our feelings, and ways to tame and prune this loop by challenging our mindset and learning to reclaim our energy to focus on healing.

Part III: Compassion examines changing the narrative and embracing your unique situation and your unique self.

Part IV: Courage explores welcoming the unexpected, gaining clarity, and stepping into wisdom.

Throughout the book, you will find quotes, personal stories, questions, and various tools that I used. There is a science and an art to healing. Science is based on what we know as true right now, and this evolves over time. The art is how we integrate science into our being and create our future. When you reach the end of each section, there are questions to reflect on. It's a good idea to write down your thoughts in a journal. Remember, it is okay if you don't have all the answers right now; you can always revisit it later. So, grab a journal, a notebook, Post-its, or a highlighter to capture the nuggets of insight that resonate with you. I have my favorite quotes on the bathroom mirror, in the car, in my Passion Planner, and anywhere I will see them daily, whether I am brushing my teeth, stopped at a light, or reflecting on my week. One of my favorite Buddhist sayings is "Pain is inevitable, but suffering is optional." This quote reminds me that I have a choice and pain doesn't have to rule my life.

You might find yourself amazed or surprised when inspiration hits, so there will be times you have to just hit the speech-to-text in your Notes app on your phone. Also, at the end of each section is a list of suggested readings to go deeper into the process. I've met many people who said they tried to read books by Dr. Joe Dispenza, which is where my journey started, but got lost in the science. After you read this book, I suggest you reread Dr. Joe's books. If you have to gloss over the technical parts, that is okay, but keep reading. You can always go back and reread it again. The more you read it or hear the concepts, the easier it will be to understand and integrate them. Although I pushed through one of his books, I didn't retain one hundred percent of the information. After reading all of his books over the past year, I'm not finished. I'm still learning and developing my understanding. I couldn't connect this type of learning with anything that I've known; this was all uncharted territory. I urge you to continue reading, learning, and experiencing the newness of this journey. What if you could trade fear, resentment, and suffering for healing?

The challenges of our lives can be viewed as a burden or an opportunity. Many times, we put the needs of others ahead of our own and push through. We embody our roles as parents, caretakers, mental health professionals, coaches, and teachers but rarely pause for self-care, or we have self-care routines that are short-lived.

By profession, I am a licensed psychologist with a degree in School-Clinical/Child Psychology, and I am an American Board of School Neuropsychology Diplomate. I work in a school setting and have a private practice. I have always trusted doctors. When I have medical concerns, I automatically call a medical specialist. I value and respect my medical team and their expertise. They have always provided a course of action, and I was always able to recover, move on, and return to "normal." With this diagnosis, I was under the care of a "pain management" doctor, and I was in another realm. I remember that I kept wanting my body to be the way it used to be as opposed to accepting how it was, but I realized those weren't my only options. The medical doctors had done their part in following the medical model; now, it was time for me to do my part. I knew I would have to dismantle the illusion of normalcy that I yearned to return to. I also knew that whatever I decided, I needed to feel it so strongly that no one else could tell me otherwise. And that is where it all started. I was a psychologist diving into her own psyche. As a "helping professional," I want to show others the path based on science, but at the same time, I want to help you realize that there is an art to healing. That art takes heart and passion. The kind of heart that would indicate you are willing to take a risk and do things differently and believe in possibility. Through this journey, I learned to create my own masterpiece. It's like the difference between being tossed around by the waves and learning to float.

My reason for writing this book is to use my voice to empower others to tap into their inner resources. Whether you are dealing with stress, chronic pain, anxiety, depression, or past trauma, there is a light at the end of the tunnel. What I have learned is that if we open up to different ways of thinking, we can change the trajectory of our lives. Like most people, I had to hit rock bottom to get to the root of my pain.

Once you finish this book, you will see yourself differently and feel energetically different. You'll discover a *you* that you can't yet imagine. Is that scary? Good. Before I began this process, I had a hard time being with myself, understanding myself, and trusting my own judgment. I was fearful of my condition worsening and losing my autonomy, and I realized these thoughts and feelings were making me feel worse. I wasn't even aware that this pain went deeper than the surface pains I was feeling. It is reported that only 5% of our mind is conscious—that means 95% is under the surface. Over time, I learned what stress feels like in my body and where it resides. Through this process, I learned to prioritize self-care and not let my temporary emotions interfere with my routine. What I learned is that I am the most important person in my life. By the end of the book, my hope is that you will feel the same about yourself.

> **"You can't pursue wisdom without being willing to get uncomfortable."**
>
> George Mumford
> *The Mindful Athlete*

Now is your time. All we have is the moment we are in <u>right now</u>. The past is done, and the future has not yet unfolded. If you have been struggling with chronic pain, stress, anxiety, depression, or past trauma (which all lead to physical disorders) and are unsure what direction to go in, this book is for you. The only way to finish is to start. The future you want is on the other side of the door. Kick that shit down. I often hear that wisdom comes with age, but that's a lie. Wisdom comes with overcoming life's challenges. It comes from integrating knowledge with experience and admitting that you didn't know it all. It's about when everything falls apart, and you are able to rise like a phoenix from the ashes and turn your test into your testimony. It doesn't come from calm waters. It comes from the storms of life. Wisdom is found when you are brought to your knees and you are praying while you brace yourself to rise up.

So, ask yourself the following questions:

- Is this a journey I want to take?

- What do I have to lose?

"We are all connected spirits and there's great power within each of us if we are willing to explore and embrace it."

Dr. Sabrina Crouch

PART I

Connection

"Inaction breeds doubt and fear. Action breeds confidence and courage..."

Dale Carnegie

CHAPTER 1

Knowledge is Power
(If You Act on It)

Knowing my Body

It was a normal, predictable day until it wasn't. I was about to have a cup of afternoon tea in my favorite mug for that pick-me-up that I needed to push through the rest of the workday and into my evening. At the time, I was enrolled in an online sport psychology certification program at JFKU. The rest of the day was already mapped out, as were the next six months, which is typical for this type A master of my own universe. I can't count how many times I've performed that same motion: reaching my hand out to pick up a coffee mug while holding the teapot in my right hand. However, this time was very different, and one thing I know very well is my body. It was like my life had changed in the blink of an eye. Each day after this brought a new, unfamiliar experience. Swelling in my fingers was one thing, but one morning, I woke up and my fingers on my left hand would not move; I panicked. I stared at them, but my brain couldn't get

3

them to move. So, instead of getting on a plane to California for vacation, I was going for an MRI.

I have played sports enough to know when I have a sprain, a tear, or a broken bone. This pain was clearly out of proportion for the situation. The MRI confirmed a diagnosis of cervical stenosis, which is when there is inflammation in the spinal canal, causing it to narrow and compress on the nerves. For me, it was C4-C5, which caused neck stiffness, nerve pain radiating down my left arm, and hypersensitivity in my fingers to changes in temperature and pressure. This was scary, but it was mostly the uncertainty that weighed on me as I contemplated how this would affect my life. My thoughts were racing, and within a short amount of time, I withdrew from classes, contemplated changing my career, selling my home, and a host of other "what if" scenarios. As the weeks went on, if my body felt good, I was happy, and if my body was hurting, I was miserable. The doctor recommended two things: epidurals and medication. I opted for the epidurals, which led to some relief, but when the pain returned, I was faced with the second option, which was medication. As I look back, I see now what this pain was costing me in terms of my relationships with others. There were times when I did not want to go out with friends, talk on the phone, or answer the question, "How are you feeling?" Although there is a physical component to pain, people rarely talk about how pain takes hold of your mind, and that was what was happening to me. I was frequently gritting my teeth, uncomfortable in my own skin, and I was unsure of my body's ability to perform the tasks that I relied on it to do. Another thing about pain that is chronic, whether physical or emotional, is that it is subjective. It is often hard to explain, and it is hard for others to understand.

What I became conscious of from this journey is our bodies are very complex, and the more we understand how they work and the influence we have over them, the better our outcomes. No one is free from stress or pain, and many things occur that throw us off balance. It is true that our bodies are designed to protect us. Imagine if there was no pain signal when you burned your finger or if a diabetic didn't realize that they had a sore on their leg. Many have heard of the fight-or-flight response. In the short-term, our bodies can adjust in response to threats or dangerous situations, but in situations of prolonged stress, we are changing our internal chemistry and impacting our genes. Although pain is subjective, chronic pain is usually defined as persistent and lasting for more than six months. One of the most important things I learned in my reading is that we can turn on the stress response by thought alone. This was powerful and a game-changer for me. So, whether we are in a stressful situation or merely thinking about a past stressor, our bodies will respond in the same way, releasing those hormones and preparing to fight. The most challenging part of the pain I was feeling was that I couldn't anticipate it or predict when it would end. So, I was triggering that stress response frequently in my body. Once you understand this, you will realize how critical it is to work on your level of self-awareness. Knowledge is power but only if you use it to improve your situation, and this requires action.

Chronic pain is one of the most common types of health problems among U.S. adults. Statistics from the Center for Disease Control, for example, indicate that chronic pain affects one in five (20 percent) of adults. This translates to more than 50 million people. There is a lot at stake, and the people who deal with chronic pain are us, our friends, mothers, fathers, grandparents, sisters, brothers, and children. The reach of the impact of chronic pain is bigger than the individual, and none of us operate in isolation. We are members of families, communities, and work environments, and how we feel impacts these relationships. This means that how we think about chronic pain and the tools we use to solve it will influence generations.

"You can believe the diagnosis, not the prognosis."

Deepak Chopra

It is important to understand that when people with chronic pain see their condition only as a medical problem, they run the risk of over-relying on medical treatments such as medication and surgeries.

I'm sure there are patients with chronic pain who obtain excellent results with medical treatments alone; however, many other patients either obtain limited improvements or resort to self-medicating with alcohol or other drugs. The more a person relies on medical approaches as their primary treatment for chronic pain symptoms, the higher their risk of experiencing these negative outcomes.

Everyone is a Google MD

How many times have you typed your symptoms into a Google search engine and came up with a possible diagnosis, prognosis, and treatment options? I do this all the time. In this age of information at our fingertips, it can be a blessing, a curse, or anything in between. Due to the abundance of accessible information, we have to practice discernment. I spent months exploring alternatives to medication. Each time I spoke to my doctor about alternative treatments, I would get "a look." Despite this, I explored alternatives anyway. I consulted with a nutritionist, a physical therapist, a chiropractor, and an acupuncturist. In the alternative medicine realm, I learned Reiki, Emotional Freedom Technique (EFT), and mindfulness-based stress reduction (MBSR). I spoke to anyone that would listen and was given dozens of suggestions such as turmeric, CBD oil, and Arnica, but I was way past that, and after a few months, I had upgraded to more medication. Most of the suggestions I received were helpful in some way in terms of shaping my perspective, but I needed something to take me further. This wasn't my first go-round with injuries and medical conditions that I have had over the years. I have had rotator cuff repairs (right and left shoulder), left shoulder arthroscopy, a torn meniscus, gluten sensitivities, gastritis, pelvic floor dysfunction, osteoarthritis, and osteopenia. All of those could be corrected or managed, but I had to wrap my brain around this new condition. I was looking to feel empowered, like I had some control, and that I was not a victim to this condition.

Becoming the Diagnosis

I've read it dozens of times in books, and as a mental health professional, I often remind clients that it is not the stress that's the problem but how you interpret the stress. So, how does this relate to chronic pain or any chronic condition? The higher the perceived stress, the more dysfunctional the pain modulation capabilities become. In other words, the type of stress and magnitude of how it is interpreted and felt in the body determines how it is manifested in the pain system. There are many factors that can contribute to a person's pain experience, including age, gender, and life experiences, but one of the most important factors is our psychological state. Perception is everything.

Let's think about how we often respond to any diagnosis, where it takes us emotionally, and how our body responds to it as we "become the diagnosis." We attach survival emotions to medical conditions, such as fear and anxiety, which feed our body chemically through the stress response. We have an image etched in our mind of what the condition looks and feels like, which we begin to embody. We become loyal to our suffering, not only in the location in our body where we feel it but also in our mind.

I'll admit it; I have read all the possible symptoms and thought, *This is me!* I have read about how the condition unfolds and wondered, *Is this what I have to look forward to?* I have played out every worst-case scenario in my head. When the doctor told me there was no cure, but once my condition worsened I would be a candidate for surgery, it left me little comfort. There can be a range of reactions to the challenge of a new or persistent condition, such as fear, despair, worry, anxiety, and, maybe, even depression. I felt them all; I call it the emotional cocktail. There's nothing wrong with these emotions as they are all typical, along with shock and surprise, but what I found is that I was remaining in these emotional states for too long, and it was changing my mood. It was almost as if the pain had its own voice, and it was louder than my thoughts. I knew I had to figure something out, or this would be the death of me. Not physically, but that my spirit would be broken. That's how strong I felt that I needed to find something to manage the pain. I started reading about using meditation to heal, and initially, I thought this couldn't be possible. I knew it would take time, but I was willing to explore and try something outside of my comfort zone.

Finding a Path

There are many myths about meditation. The ones I believed and often heard were:

1. *I have to sit still.* The reality is you can sit, stand, walk, or lie down while meditating.

2. *I have to stop my thoughts.* This is an impossible feat, and trying to accomplish this will only lead to frustration. What meditation focuses on is slowly shifting our attention. I started out by focusing on my breath and the rise and fall of my chest as my breathing relaxed. I also cut out as much external stimuli as possible by using noise-canceling headphones. If for some reason my mind drifted—making a grocery list or recalling a conversation from earlier in the day—then once I realized it, I gently brought myself back to my breath.

3. *This is a spiritual or religious practice that goes against my religion.* Meditation is about quieting the noise in our minds. It doesn't require a spiritual practice. I know many Christians who utilize both prayer and meditation. Prayer is speaking to God, and meditation is waiting for the response. Remember, there are many different types of meditation, so look into the philosophy behind the method you are considering.

4. *I don't have enough time.* The bottom line is people make time for what's important to them. If you believe you don't have time, then meditation is not important enough for you to try. More importantly, it is not about the quantity; it is about the quality of the time. I started off with five minutes, and after a few months, I worked my way up to an hour. When I meditated, I found a different realm and a different state where I was not worried about time. I found a state of peace,

flow, and oneness with my breath. My mind and body were in sync, and sensing that what I was doing was working helped me stick to this new routine.

After reading *Breaking the Habit of Being Yourself* and trying one of the meditations (halfheartedly, I'll admit), I decided to read one of Dr. Joe Dispenza's other books, *Becoming Supernatural*, and something clicked. What attracted me to the work of Dr. Joe Dispenza was the combination of neuroscience, psychoneuroimmunology, and spirituality. This combination exposed a whole new world for me. A world of epigenetics, neuroplasticity, and quantum physics. They were all new ideas, but the most important part was that I was open to learning and growing. I knew very few people who practiced meditation, at least this method. Initially, friends I spoke with looked at me with a *this chick is crazy* expression. I did have a few open-minded friends who were supportive, but more importantly, I connected with people who were on a similar path through groups on Facebook and at live events. I believe that just because you haven't experienced something on your journey, it doesn't mean other people's experiences are wrong. Don't let anyone deny your reality based on their experiences. The tools and practices that I discovered were a perfect match for me, and I urge you to explore different methods and find what works best for you. For me, it wasn't only about the book *Becoming Supernatural,* but how I was able to bring the meditations to life by integrating them into my being. I often get asked, "Does meditation work?" The only response I can give is, "What are you willing to do to create the life that you say you want?"

Managing My Mind

When starting a new routine, your body has to adjust, and it will respond with attempts to revert back to a familiar state. It's just like it is at the start of a new year, when everyone makes that resolution, and the gym is packed for the first month. We all know what happens after that. For me, a few days into meditating, I realized that I was having what I call "side effects." When I sat down, my skin would itch, my body would feel hot and then cold, and then the big one—nausea—as my energy moved through my body. These were all distractions, and luckily, I did not give in, and the itchiness and nausea went away. Don't be alarmed; I wasn't. But it did make me curious. After this experience, I spoke to my Reiki friend Samantha who indicated that it was energy that was blocked and released, and that is simply what it felt like.

Just know that whatever you feel that makes you uncomfortable through this process is most likely a DISTRACTION. The key is to push past the discomfort. Once you do, your body will adjust, and these distractions will go away. If this talk of energy moving through your body and energy centers makes you uncomfortable, good. I was once there as well until I started feeling it moving and was able to focus my attention on a part of my body and sense it in this way. Where attention goes, energy flows.

"Never limit yourself because of others' limited imaginations. If you adopt their attitudes, then the possibility won't exist because you'll have already shut it out. You can hear other people's wisdom, but you've got to re-evaluate the world for yourself."

Dr. Mae Jemison
The first black woman to travel into space

A few weeks into meditating, I was feelin' myself (in my Beyonce voice), and I thought I had mastered my mind. I decided that I was ready to resume my exercise class after feeling like my pain was under control with medication, meditation, and reduced physical activity. I thought I was ready. As I started on the bike, I felt a familiar sensation in my wrist, and in my mind, this was how the painful nerve sensations of the past always started. It didn't take long for me to become panicked and fearful that it was coming back. At that moment, I was predicting my pain based on my past, which meant that subconsciously I felt that the pain was inevitable. It took me a few minutes to settle my mind down and realize that it was only a sensation and not the pain. I was still checking for the pain, which meant I still had a lot more work to do. Clearly, these skills did not yet carry over to other aspects of my life, but I was confident I was on the right track. Just because I found a path, it doesn't mean that there weren't bumps along the way.

Tough Questions

I was looking for direction, but I was led to insight. I recalled how helpful my guide was on a trip to Egypt. I was experiencing sinus pain and congestion. My guide told me to stop taking medicine, and he would take me to a shop for all-natural healing products. We ended up in an oil shop and a man brought me a small cup with hot water and a few drops of mint oil to inhale. I have been doing this since 2018 and have not taken any prescription or over-the-counter medication for sinusitis since. I wondered if my guide Alaa could help me with this new challenge. We spoke over the phone, and I explained my symptoms. Alaa asked me, "What is the cause of your pain?" I quickly said that it was a car accident. He replied, "No." His next question would be more profound. He asked me, "What are you holding on to that you need to get rid of?" At the time, I had no response. Initially, it felt like he dropped a bomb, but as I reflected on it, it was more like he planted a seed, and unexpectedly, I would see the answer sprouting into the light. Developing a new relationship with yourself takes time. I was always willing to invest in my professional development, and now, I was investing in my personal development. When I spoke to Alaa months later, he told me straight out, "Whatever is bothering you, let that shit go." This time he was giving it to me straight, and his message was understood.

As you think about your own situation, only you know what you have been through, and there's so much more out of conscious awareness. Now look in the mirror and ask yourself, "What am I holding on to that I need to get rid of?" It may take time before the answer is revealed, but trust the process.

CHAPTER 2

Recalibrating

I have always had a love for sports, whether it was tennis, track, or basketball. It was not only about the physical training of athletes but also the mind of the athlete that intrigued me. They have the minds of warriors. When everything fell apart for me, I was studying sport psychology and learning how to work with athletes to improve their performance. You often hear coaches say the game is 90% mental and 10% physical. I began to wonder how I could apply this knowledge to my present challenge. So, my new sport was meditation—90% mental, 10% physical. It would require me to learn how to self-regulate by learning how to be still, focus on my breathing, and get into heart and brain coherence, which I will discuss later in this chapter.

"Through the portals of silence, the healing sun of wisdom and peace will shine upon you."

Paramahansa Yogananda

Pleasure in the Pause

Stillness seems elusive in these challenging times; it feels like there is always something to do or something going on that we may miss. We are competing with not only the distractions of the external world but also the internal chatter of our internal world—things to do and reminders that keep us attached to the past or the future. We often overlook the only moment we truly have, and that is the present. This moment right now. Ryan Holiday, in his book *Stillness is the Key,* said, "Stillness is the key to unlocking all we are capable of."

When was the last time you turned off the television, turned off notifications, turned your phone off, or put it on *do not disturb?* Even I have my guilty pleasures. Technology can be addicting, and it can change our neurological wiring, but small adjustments can lead to creating new habits. When you can quiet your external and internal worlds, you can become a master and find pleasure in the pause.

What is the present moment? The present moment is the gift we've been given right now, not the moments of the past or the thoughts of the future. It's being with ourselves, and this is challenging for many. It is learning to be alone but not feel lonely. Cultivating stillness is a skill, just like many things we have had to learn. We have to be purposeful, disciplined, responsible, and make a choice to reclaim the present moment one minute, and sometimes one second, at a time. Although society may steer us in one direction, we have to learn how to direct ourselves and become selective about our input.

How do we access the present moment? We have to ask ourselves, *Is this use of energy in alignment with my values and purpose?* We have to decide what is nice rather than what is necessary. This is easier said than done, but this is the choice we must make moment to moment in order to reclaim the time we need to be still and connect with our inner selves. Only you can decide what's best for you, but be sure to choose actions that will empower you. This process will allow you to regain your most important commodities: your time and energy. These are the two things you need to conserve and channel inward because that is where the healing begins.

We all have things that we enjoy doing and maybe some fear of missing out (FOMO). I have my "guilty pleasures," such as listening to the Breakfast Club or binge-watching a series, but I know that I have to limit these and recalibrate. So, how do I do it? For every activity that comes before me, I ask myself, *Is it necessary?* You have to believe you have a choice. It has nothing to do with what others want or expect from you but what you want and expect for yourself. I remember my guide, Alaa, telling me, "You are the most important person in this life." Now, I want you to say it; "I am the most important person in this life."

"Without full awareness of breathing, there can be no development of meditative stability and understanding."

Thich Nhat Hanh

B-R-E-A-T-H-E

The breath is the center of our life. For centuries, Eastern medicine has focused on controlling this physiological response through practice. I remember one of the first books I bought as a graduate student in psychology was *The Relaxation Response* by Herbert Benson, which described the mind-body connection and identified ways to self-regulate. Breath is where it all starts.

We breathe automatically, without thought, but I am talking about an intentional deep breath. One of the first things I needed to retrain myself in, in order to be able to increase the amount of time I was able to sit and meditate, was taking relaxed deep breaths. It had been years since I had been diving, but relaxed breathing is the key to not rapidly depleting your oxygen. I remember learning how to control my exhale in a slow manner. It was all coming back to me.

There are many different breathing techniques. I found that techniques that encourage counting are great place to start, but for me, counting kept me in my head, and the goal for me was to get out of that cerebral space. I found that diaphragmatic breathing, also known as belly breathing, was helpful because it encouraged me to refocus my attention on my body. I know integrating new strategies can be overwhelming, but let's focus on the process, not the end result. Any attempt is a victory, so the pressure is off.

Belly Breathing Instructions

- Lie on your back on a flat surface (or in bed) with your knees bent. You can use a pillow under your head and your knees for support if that's more comfortable.

- Place one hand on your upper chest and the other on your belly, just below your rib cage.

- Breathe in slowly through your nose, letting the air in deeply, towards your lower belly. The hand on your chest should remain still, while the one on your belly should rise.

- Tighten your abdominal muscles and let them fall inward as you exhale through pursed lips. The hand on your belly should move down to its original position.

You can also practice this sitting in a chair with your knees bent and your shoulders, head, and neck relaxed. Practice for five to ten minutes several times a day, if possible. Belly breathing has many benefits, including stress relief, providing oxygen to your cells, and improving concentration, and most importantly, it doesn't cost anything. However, you have to decide if you are worth the time and effort.

The greatest benefit of belly breathing is achieving deep relaxation. However, I also want you to understand the science behind it. Bringing your breath up from your belly, as opposed to focusing on higher regions, works by stimulating the parasympathetic nervous system, which slows down our systems, evoking the feeling of relaxation. The more you practice it, the easier it will get. I remember going on a dive and not being told ahead of time that we would swim through a cave. Talk about shallow breathing. I was underwater hyperventilating, using up all my oxygen. In that moment, I had to focus and slow down my breathing and keep that oxygen flowing to my cells, and then I was able to clear my mind. Many guided meditations, like the ones that I follow, start with a breathing technique; breathwork calms the mind and evokes a positive feeling of connection between the mind and body by slowing down those brain waves.

Once you master belly breathing then you can explore other breathing techniques that involve elongated breaths and holding your breath to stimulate your nervous system. These yoga breathing techniques are the key to boosting your immune system as well as calming your nervous system and slowing down brain waves to Delta. This brain wave state is where many believe they will be able to access the unconscious mind (don't knock it until you try it). Remember, this process is about exploring alternatives that you may not have considered.

Heart and Brain Coherence

By now, you may be thinking, *What is the point of stillness and focus breathing?* It's all about achieving heart and brain coherence. Basically, stress throws our bodies off balance. When stressed, there is a feeling, hormonal response, and physiological response. For example, when anxious, worried, or frustrated, there is an increase in cortisol levels, and our heart rhythm becomes incoherent. On the other end of the spectrum, when feeling positive emotions, such as gratitude, DHEA levels increase, and our heart rhythms become coherent. So, the objective is to interrupt this stress response and bring our hearts into coherence. When you're in low coherence, you're activating your limbic brain, which is driven by fight, flight, and freeze responses; while in high coherence, you're activating your frontal lobe in the front part of your brain and accessing your thinking and reasoning abilities. Coherence is important to avoid your brain being hijacked by your emotions. Have you ever been so locked into your emotions that you were unable to think straight? I have been there. I always say you can't rationalize with an irrational person, and this is exactly why. Their brain has been hijacked. Like any new skill, this will take practice, but it only takes a few minutes a day. Remember, any step you take toward this goal is a victory.

Heart Math Institute has a quick coherence technique that involves you focusing your attention on your heart area and imagining your breath is flowing in and out. In addition, focusing on a positive feeling, such as gratitude, can help you slow down your breathing and breathe deeply. This is a research-based method that you can use to reduce the impact of stress on your body. Heart Math also has practitioners and trainers who have studied their methods. They can assist with working through a variety of concerns such as depression, anxiety, and ADHD.

> *"When we are in heart and brain coherence we can harmonize and optimize our human potential."*
>
> Gregg Braden

Why Focus on the Heart?

Researchers at Heart Math Institute have found that the heart sends signals 5,000 times stronger to the brain than the brain sends to the heart, suggesting that the more you focus on your heart, the easier you will be able to transform your stress response in your brain. In addition, as you learn to shift the signals going to the heart, you can create new patterns that the brain will remember. This makes the heart a powerful organ. It also emits a field of energy up to 8–10 feet wide. Your heart can not only transform stress but also it can build resilience. Once you cultivate resilience, you can access it on demand. All it takes is a willingness to go through the process of increasing awareness to shift attitudes and change old habits. Remember, we are not focusing on the outside situations that are out of our control; we are trying to master our inner world. This is a more long-lasting solution to stress than alcohol, retail therapy, vacations, spa visits, and time off work.

When was the last time you tuned in to your own energy or someone else's energy? Once you're able to regulate, it will be easier to tune in to your own energy, know what you're feeling, and easily discern the energy of others. Have you ever heard of the phrase "energy is contagious"? One of the side effects of learning these techniques is that you may no longer resonate with others in the same way because you feel different energetically. I used to overlook this in my interactions with others, but now I realize that the strongest energy I want to sense is my own. As I started to tune in to how I felt, I noticed that I was more selective about the energy around me. I disengaged from people and situations for periods of time, and as I re-engaged, I sensed how it felt for me. If it didn't feel like it was in alignment with what I valued and my purpose, I unapologetically released it. I do believe that people are capable of change, so occasionally, I would increase the frequency of engagement to see if I sensed more order and harmony.

Technology

Instead of being consumed by technology, let's use it to our advantage. If you are like me and you enjoy technology, it is important to be selective. There are a few websites, tools, and apps that I have been using regularly, and I am sure that as time goes on, I will discover more. I highly recommend the Heart Math Inner Balance Monitor, which I have been using for about a year. This was essential for me as I learned to sit for longer meditations. The Inner Balance Monitor is my favorite self-regulation tool for myself and I highly recommend it for others. In working with coaching clients, it allows me to monitor their progress in between sessions.

The Inner Balance Monitor clips on to your ear and syncs with the Inner Balance phone app. The monitor analyzes and displays heart rhythm, measured by Heart Rate Variability (HRV), which indicates how emotional states are affecting our nervous system. It also provides immediate feedback through sound, coaches you as you practice, and tracks your progress over time. It is helpful to look back and see my coherence levels when I first started as compared to where I am now. Research has shown that a few minutes of daily practice can reduce and prevent the negative effects of stress, such as overwhelm, fatigue and exhaustion, sleep disruption, anxiety, and burnout. After practicing for only five minutes twice a day for a week, I noticed two things. First, when I focused on my breathing and the sensations of my breath moving in and out of my body, I wasn't focused on my pain. Second, I was able to tune in to places of tension within my body and then target those areas to release it. The first step in learning to meditate is to be able to focus on your breath. For more information, go to www.heartmath.com.

One of my newer discoveries is Muse. Once I started meditating and felt physical changes in my body, I was curious as to what my brain measurements would show. Muse is a brain-sensing headband that syncs to an app that will track your progress and provide feedback as you meditate. It also tracks EEG, heart rate, body movement, and breathing. The first time I used it, I didn't read the instructions, and I wondered why, at times, I heard thunderstorms, which I found annoying. At other times, there were birds chirping. It just so happens that this is how this technology works, and it provides feedback based on whether your mind is calm or active; thunderstorms indicated my mind was very active, and the birds chirping meant I was in the zone. Some lessons are learned through trial and error, which is fine. For more information, check out their website www.choosemuse.com.

My other new favorite, which I was introduced to at the School Neuropsychology Conference, is Brain Tap, which combines tones and light pulses that send signals to your brain and guide you into deep relaxation. It has been known to provide maximum results in the least amount of time. It looks like a space-age headset. This research-based technology has been known to reduce mind chatter, enhance productivity, memory, focus, creativity, and provide more energy, in addition to relaxation and promoting restorative sleep. They have short but effective meditations that are very soothing. Dr. Patrick Porter also does live meditations on Wednesdays that you can find on their social media page. Their website is www.braintap.com.

Recently, I began training in neurofeedback. Although I am looking forward to using it to help others, I am starting with myself. Neurofeedback involves mapping the brain and looking for areas of over- or under-activity. Eventually, I will be training my own brain. This is just another tool I am using to gain awareness of my functioning. I look forward to using neuroscience to improve the brain health of people who would not typically have access to this type of training.

I am sure there are lots of other technologies and apps out there to assist you on your journey; you just need to find what works best for you. Some of the other strategies that I use to ensure that I maximize my time include using a calendar app with alarms, turning off notifications and alerts during focus time, putting my phone on do not disturb, limiting television to one hour a day, wearing noise-canceling headphones (you would be surprised how good these work), and soothing music such as jazz, classical, binaural beats, or a white noise machine. When I speak of recalibrating, I'm referring to using stillness, your breath, and heart by tapping into those centers in your body that can connect with your brain to change your reaction to pain, fear, and anxiety. Once you start settling yourself down, observing yourself, and attending inward, you can recalibrate your internal settings to be comfortable with stillness. Then you will hear your inner voice sing, just as I did. Inside yourself is where your intuition lies, and that is a powerful place to be.

Reflections

1. Proper breathing techniques are key to being able to regulate the body and slow down the mind.

2. Changing the heart and brain's rhythmic patterns can provide feedback to increase self-awareness and consciousness resulting in intentional and longer-lasting changes.

3. We can use technology to our advantage instead of being consumed by it. Technology can be used to provide us with feedback and monitor whether we're on the right track.

4. It's important to ask yourself questions. Not just how or why, but what. What are you holding on to that you need to get rid of?

Go Deeper

Breathe by Belisa Vranich

Stillness is the Way by Ryan Holiday

The Body Keeps the Score by Bessel Van Der Kolk, MD

The Wim Hof Method by Wim Hof, Elissa Epel, PhD

https://www.heartmath.org/

PART II

Clarity

"I discovered that we can only find peace in the present, and the present moment is all we really have."

Dr. Sabrina Crouch

CHAPTER 3

The Power of Thoughts and Feelings

Everything that we've discussed so far sounds great in an ideal world, but eventually, you are going to have to come to terms with your inner thoughts and feelings and how those interact with others. What happens then? Let's dive into thoughts and feelings. Brain scientist Jill Bolte Taylor reported the average time it takes for an emotion to move through the nervous system is 90 seconds. Wow! What keeps fueling those emotions are our thoughts. Once we're able to slow down the automaticity of this thought-feeling connection, we can find the right place to jump off. Because so many thoughts are unconscious, we need to be aware and gain clarity as to which thoughts and feelings we want to foster and which ones we want to tame or prune.

As we interact with others, we often encounter differences of opinion, as each person is stuck in their own way of thinking. You know those conversations with friends or coworkers that seem to go nowhere? When those types of conversations happen, our egos keep us locked-in. We want to be right. We want the other person to hear our point of view, and we are frustrated when that doesn't happen. Once again, you have to decide. Is this a battle worth fighting? For me, I ask myself, *Do I want to be right, or do I want to be free?* About 95% of the time, I choose freedom. The times when I get stuck in wanting to be right, I have to ask myself, *Will this debate matter a week from now, a month from now, or a year from now?* If not, then I have to let it go. Remember, people's opinions typically reflect their level of comfort based on their past and usually indicate what they would do if they were you, but they are not.

Sometimes, people's opinions will resonate with you, and other times, they will not. If you're trying to get into a new zone mentally, you have to be aware of this. This is not about judging; you have a choice. For as many people as you know, you can have that many opinions. Typically, when someone starts off with, "You should," "You must," "You ought to," or, "You have to," my brain immediately shuts off to what they have to say afterward. If I said these words to myself in my head, I would be using guilt to shape my decision. I find that I now gravitate towards people who, when giving advice, say, "You may want to," or, "It would be helpful to," or people who are willing to ask me questions to process instead of trying to "give me an answer." At some point, you have to make a decision for yourself. You can welcome other people's ideas, but don't let them hold power over you. When I was first diagnosed with stenosis and started sharing with others about my struggles, many people meant well but often had trouble finding the right words to say in response. It is especially hard for people when someone does not "look like" they have a condition.

When you're dealing with your own condition and caring for others in some way—whether it's your children, parents, or providing emotional support to friends—you're going to need to make space for yourself. This will involve setting boundaries with others. I know people have mixed feelings about boundaries, but I believe boundaries equal self-love. At times, we have difficulty setting them, but this usually reflects our own fears, guilt, or self-doubt. It's a process, and it is one that I'm still working on. One of the first steps to setting boundaries is being clear about what you value, and if someone crosses it, you need to be able to communicate that in a way that's direct. Boundaries reflect your level of self-confidence. You have permission to say "no" unapologetically. We teach people how to treat us.

The Science of Thoughts

Laboratory of Neuro-Imaging reports that the average person experiences 70,000 thoughts per day, the running commentary that some call mental chatter. That's right, they are often about worst-case scenarios (what can go wrong), past mistakes and regrets (what did go wrong), and predictions for the future (what will go wrong). Most of these thoughts aren't conscious, which means our subconscious mind is running the show. Your subconscious determines the lens that you see the world through, which is based on your experiences and interpretation of those experiences. It is also influenced by other sources (friends, social media, news, fake news, etc.). Freud compared the power of the mind to an iceberg. The tip above water is the conscious mind (5–10%), and the subconscious mind is the rest of the iceberg that is submerged (90–95%). The bottom line is there is a lot under the surface that we haven't even explored within ourselves. This is not always a comfortable place for many, which is why there are therapists and other professionals to facilitate the process of going deeper. We can't address what we don't see; this is why awareness is so important. This process starts with us, and we have a lot riding on this. Our mental health is the mental health of our families, and our family health is the health of our communities, which in turn provides an opportunity for communities to reclaim their power and rewrite the narrative. With increased self-awareness, we are in a better position to not only advocate for ourselves with our personal health issues but also apply our knowledge to the social and political concerns of our communities.

There are many subconscious thinking patterns that we can get caught up in. Relating to your condition, whether it be physical or emotional pain, what are you telling yourself? In his book, *Change Your Brain Change Your Life*, Dr. Daniel Amen says it is important to identify your automatic negative thoughts (ANTs). He identified 9 that are common. The first 6 are:

1. **All or nothing:** Categorizing something as all good or all bad. For example, one slip up, and you are ready to throw it all away.

2. **"Always" thinking:** Keywords to look out for are *always* and *never*. This leads to overgeneralizations.

3. **Focusing on the negative:** What you see magnifies. If you only see the negative, then you neglect any positive aspects of the situation.

4. **Thinking with our feelings:** For example, I used to think *My condition is never going to improve!*

5. **Guilt beating:** This includes words like "should," "must", "ought to," and "have to."

6. **Labeling:** Calling yourself or someone else a negative name. It is almost like you are defeated before you even begin.

Additionally, there are 3 that he calls the red ants. They are the ones that really get us. These are **fortune-telling**—predicting worst-case scenarios. I can raise my hand here. **Mind-reading** is when you think you know what someone else is thinking and respond to what you think they are thinking when they have not said a word. Then there is **blame**—when you don't take responsibility for your success or lack thereof. If you fall into this trap, you be playing the role of victim without even realizing it.

Seeing Red

It's not just the story we tell ourselves, it is the meaning and emotion we give to the story and how we have internalized it without awareness. So, let's say we have a memory of a traumatic situation. There's the memory and the story that we attach to it that we carry with us with all of its emotion. If we close our eyes we can sense it and be right back in that space. When I started meditating regularly, I would wake up the next morning recalling the same memory from when I was a child. These memories did not scare me. I would say that I was more curious about why they were coming up and what that meant.

One of my earliest memories as a child was when I was in the hospital after having my tonsils removed. I vividly remember waking up, choking on blood, and being rushed back to the operating room with the bright lights overhead. I remember how the nurses put ice cubes in my mouth, and I was spitting them out covered in blood. When color is introduced, it relates to emotions. For me, the intensity of the color red signified a past injury. I recently decided to ask my mother about the accuracy of these memories, which I had never had the courage to do. It turns out that I was actually only three years old when this happened, which speaks even more powerfully to how trauma gets imprinted on the brain consciously or unconsciously.

I would say as a child, I was relatively quiet, often silent, and this carried over into adulthood. For most of my life, I felt like my voice didn't matter or, at times, like I didn't have a voice. I felt that both my voice and my body were fragile. This is the story I had been carrying with me. Now, I am an adult and aware of this subconscious belief that I was weak, and I am facing the challenge of how to manage and make sense of this pain. The great thing about becoming aware is that I can now challenge my subconscious beliefs. It all returned to that profound question Alaa asked me, and I think I found an answer. I can now hug my inner three-year-old, tell her she is safe, and release her. This was just one layer; most of us have multiple layers of trauma.

You can't fix what you don't see. Trauma doesn't always have to lead to being traumatized. Some of us have had life-threatening trauma, and no one is exempt from the trauma of emotional or stressful events, but feeling traumatized can lead to long-lasting emotional and behavioral challenges. Traces of trauma are imprinted in our brain, body, and mind and can be reactivated and triggered at any time. I know from my own EEG brain map that I also have traces of trauma. I don't respond to this with fear but with curiosity. This knowledge doesn't have to be debilitating but can be empowering, and I can use it to my advantage. I can now play an active role in my own treatment.

Reducing the Emotion

Through the process of stillness, I was able to welcome this memory and make peace with it. Since that time, I read a book by Dr. Patrick Porter called *Awaken the Genius*. He describes a technique for removing the color of memories and calls it "shifting filters." Dr. Porter describes our perception as a filtering system and says that we can shift these perceptions by recalling an unhappy time and removing the color from the images (fading the color into black and white) or, on the flipside, recalling a happy time and adding color to those images. Our inner dialogue is powerful, and with intention, we can shape and prune it. Regarding this pain condition, I realized that by feeling anger, fear, and powerlessness, I was hating and fearing a part of myself. This pain was within me and a part of me, whether I liked it or not. I can't say "pain sucks" because pain does have a function, and it was up to me to figure out what this pain signified.

With my own situation, I realized that classifying thoughts and emotions as "good" or "bad" was limited thinking. All emotions are energy and have a vibrational frequency. One of the most helpful ways of classifying emotions that I have found is Abraham Hicks's emotional guidance scale. She divides emotions into three categories:

1. **High-feeling vibrational emotions** are positive feelings that you need to create the life that you love. These feelings include joy, freedom, appreciation, passion, hopefulness, and gratitude.

2. **Transitory emotions** are in the middle, and you can either move up or down from this state to high vibration or heavy

emotions. These include boredom, frustration, disappointment, and doubt.

3. **Heavy emotions** are often more difficult to lift yourself out of. These include worry, anger, jealousy, insecurity, fear, and powerlessness.

Remember, it's not only the words but also the feeling that is attached to the words. I had to learn to be more mindful of the words I use to describe how I'm feeling. For example, in a situation where I was disappointed, I used to describe myself as feeling devastated. Consider the imagery if someone told you they were devastated. What do you imagine? I imagine a flattened terrain with no sign of survivors. In contrast, disappointment may trigger images of a person bent over, but not down and out. Think of how much longer it would take to recover from devastation versus disappointment. Being able to change your automatic thought and feeling patterns is not easy. Initially, it can make your body feel uncomfortable. Thoughts and feelings create chemical reactions in our body, so it's important to be aware of what we're creating and recreating within with these heavier emotional patterns. The goal is to break our addiction to lower vibration, heavy, survival emotions. We can visit that emotional state, but we can't stay.

Taming the Internal Bully

We often hear about the power of positive thinking. You can read affirmations all day, but if you don't believe them, they are a waste of time. I'm not only talking about your conscious beliefs; it's those unconscious beliefs that run the show. So, why should we focus on higher vibrational feelings? Feelings such as gratitude, optimism, joy, and love can change our internal chemistry as our bodies create more feel-good chemicals. It is unrealistic to think that we can stay in high vibrational feelings all the time, but it's important to be aware of our default setting and attempt to shift the balance. Through this process, I found that being grateful regardless of my situation transformed my outlook. This was true not only regarding my medical condition but also translated to other situations in my life and improved my relationships with others.

I realized that I attracted people who were where I was emotionally. I'm owning it. I was insecure, judgmental, jealous, and fearful. As I became more conscious of my thoughts, I stopped complaining about my diagnosis, and I changed the words that I used to describe it. I also limited the time spent complaining or listening to others complain (a.k.a. the two-minute pity party) and found a like-minded tribe. I became more purposeful and selective in choosing friends. I noticed once I stopped complaining, I attracted fewer complainers. I no longer base closeness on physical proximity, such as them being family, I knew them from childhood, or I work with them. Qualities that I look for include people who are willing to step outside of their comfort zone, people who are growth-focused and open-minded. I became more protective of my energy and discovered people who were more in alignment with where I was, what I valued, and my purpose. I found connected spirits when I was guided more by my intuition than what was popular.

In learning to tame your own inner bully, you have an opportunity to examine your own subconscious beliefs and put them through the test. Especially in times dominated by social media, the origin of our beliefs may not always be clear. *The Work* by Byron Katie is helpful in examining and processing belief patterns. She calls The Work a form of meditation. On her website www.thework.com she has downloadable forms with exercises. Unless we can recognize and pause our automatic thoughts, we will only continue to reinforce these bonds. Ask yourself the following questions about your beliefs:

- Where do they come from?
- Are they true?
- How can I absolutely know they are true?
- How does my body react to my thoughts?

- Do I want to continue believing this, and if so, what purpose would it serve?

- What is it costing me to hold on to these beliefs? Intimacy? Adventure? Opportunities? Freedom?

"Feelings come and go like clouds in a windy sky. Conscious breathing is my anchor."

Thich Nhat Hanh

CHAPTER 4

Past, Present, Future ...
The Do-Have-Be Model

In the previous chapters, I discussed the importance of self-knowledge, recognizing where your thoughts and feelings originate and understanding how they can impact your condition. As human beings, we have the potential to recall information from our past (whether accurately or inaccurately) as well as envision our future. This is a superpower only humans have, and we can use this to our detriment or our advantage.

Where am I—Past, Present, or Future?

I can't count the number of times I sat and replayed past scenarios in my head. Where did it get me? Nowhere! And those worries about the future worst-case scenarios were also time drainers. They took time away from the only moment that I have—the present. There is no need to regret this. I think you only regret things if you have not learned a lesson from them. As I began to refocus my energy and learn to self-regulate, I found that I was not only able to be more present for myself but also realized this was extending into other areas of my life.

Over the past few months, it's gotten easier to spend more time in the now. I used to overlook the present by focusing on the future, but now, it's embraced. In the world of self-help and various holistic methods, you often hear where you place your attention is where you place your energy or where attention goes energy flows. One of the goals of this work is to reclaim your energy, not only from other people and external factors but also from yourself. Spending too much time concerned with the past or the future is taking it away from your present self. We always have a choice. We can't change our past, and our future is not yet here, but in the present moment, we have an opportunity.

What I discovered was that during meditation, when my focus was not on the past or future but on the now, I was able to have unexpected experiences such as energy shifting within my body and sensing energy around me. I was beginning to extend the boundaries of what I thought was possible and my body was welcoming it. In order to exert more conscious influence over my life, I had to learn how to be with myself, without all the internal and external chatter. My philosophy on life had to shift.

"If you must look back, do so forgivingly. If you must look forward, do so prayerfully. However, the wisest thing you can do is be present in the present. Gratefully."

Maya Angelou

The Unexpected Shift

When I was in my twenties, I was focused on Do-Have-Be. For me, it was going to school and working in order to have what I wanted, and this was going to make me happy, secure, etc. I thought that working and making money in order to have the house, the car, the trips, and other niceties would make me feel content. I also focused on Have-Do-Be. I thought that having the title of doctor would provide me with opportunities that would lead to me being successful. In both of these models, it was a continuous cycle of seeking more externally and never feeling like it was enough. Learning to manage chronic pain through meditation has subtly shifted the order to Be-Have-Do. This model has been used in organizational leadership. One's state of being drives influence. I love how it encourages individuals to learn to gain influence over one's own life. In order to achieve my goal of overcoming my medical disorder, I had to first ask myself, *Who do I need to be in order to accomplish this goal? What do I need to do in order to accomplish this goal? What do I need to have in order to accomplish this goal?* Surprisingly, the answers were within my own body. If I could learn to be still, present and regulate my breathing and internal systems, I could discover or uncover a level of peace. What this boiled down to was me taking personal responsibility for my situation and the outcome. This wouldn't be a one-time discovery; I would have to learn to find it in the midst of everyday life and challenges.

I have always had a "make it happen" attitude. We get these messages from various places, even my Apple watch reminds me to "make it happen" and close those exercise rings. This had always worked for me in the past to achieve various types of goals. Unfortunately, it could not be applied to my medical condition, and continuing to maintain this attitude left me frustrated. It was like trying to fit a square peg into a round hole. Making it happen doesn't work for meditation, in the sense that you can't force it. That formula doesn't work when learning to self-regulate. I sensed something had to shift in order for me to find relief. Our beliefs are usually within our range of emotional acceptance and I felt my range expanding. Once again, I was reminded of Alaa's question about the cause of my pain, and also, I was wondering about the role of my pain as it continued for months.

"If we always choose comfort, we never learn the deepest capabilities of our mind and body."

Wim Hof

Lessons in Being

Growing up, I don't recall any instruction in being. Growing up in the '70s, there were fewer external distractions and different types of distractions. We weren't competing with 24-hour news and television or technology that allowed us to interact with others across the globe. As I started college, I was caught up in being busy and working toward my personal goals. In my twenties, I didn't even think of being still, but as life does, it presented me with challenges. For me it was my father's illness. I remember my father being sick on and off for years after he was diagnosed with congestive heart failure. One day, I asked him, "What do you want me to do?" His reply was simply stated, "Just be here." It was a reminder that neither of us had control, and I couldn't fix his medical situation. I had to allow him to make decisions about his health and support him on his journey. It was a hard lesson to learn in that decade of my life to *just be*. Little did I realize that was only the beginning of my lessons in being.

On the morning of March 22, 1997, I sensed something different when I woke up. The house was eerily quiet. The dog was not moving around like usual. I've been told that some people are more intuitive than others, and I never thought I was until that moment. This was the first time I remember sensing someone's spirit. I knew in that moment that my father had died. I prepared to walk into the room to face what I already knew. The pain of knowing was indescribable. I had never experienced such profound sadness, and sensing it felt like a burden. I blocked out the sense of intuition that I felt for years and once again went back to doing. I made myself busy. The week after the funeral, I received an acceptance letter to the doctoral program, and it would be years before I paused to be with myself again. The pause was never intentional; it was always an injury that slowed me down. The stillness gave me a different sense. If I didn't make drastic changes, it would be the death of my spirit. I don't know what it was that brought me to this realization, but I knew I had to change my life. The thing about big decisions is that once you find the courage to take that step, it can translate to other areas of your life. If I could reevaluate my marriage, then I could examine all of my relationships with friends and the stuff that filled my life. This was my first big shift, and I sensed that there had to be more to life than I knew.

I started seeking different experiences, and at a Jack Kornfield workshop on Buddhist meditation, I found a connection to the past. I never thought of meditation as having the potential to heal the heart, but then he asked, "Do you know that feeling when you sense someone's spirit leaving their body?" I couldn't anticipate or contain the tears. I had never heard anyone talk about a deeper connection in such a way, and then it became clear; we are all connected spirits. For fourteen years, I felt burdened by sensing my father's spirit, and I was finally able to grieve, let go, and reinterpret it as a blessing. It was a reminder that the spirit and consciousness are not limited to this body. And what could be more powerful than that? This felt like a step away from fear and a step towards faith. Accepting my father's spirit was the beginning of me accepting my own, and an unexpected journey was unfolding. I had been so hung up on the physical nature of myself and others that I didn't acknowledge that there is a spiritual world. The crack in my heart didn't signify brokenness but many places for light to shine through.

This was another step outside of my comfort zone. That doesn't mean that I never went back to my "make it happen" default setting. Like any other skill, I would have to intentionally spend more time in this space of being so that it would become my "now" normal. With increased intentionality, synchronicities began to appear.

"Learning lessons is a little like reaching maturity. You're not suddenly more happy, wealthy, or powerful, but you understand the world around you better, and you're at peace with yourself. Learning life's lessons is not about making your life perfect, but about seeing life as it was meant to be."

Elisabeth Kubler-Ross

I know you can think of situations when you were in a Do-Have-Be or Have-Be-Do instead of Be-Have-Do. Don't be hard on yourself. When you know better, you have an opportunity to do better. We often have to repeat life lessons. No worries, there is always another opportunity. The universe will give you what you need. You just have to pay attention and realize there were times you had it all wrong.

Reflections

1. Scientist Jill Bolte Taylor indicated that the average time it takes for an emotion to move to the nervous system is 90 seconds. What keeps fueling the emotions are our thoughts. WOW!!!

2. We can only change what we're conscious of. Once you begin to slow down and engage in focused breathing, you'll be able to address the mental chatter.

3. You have an opportunity to put your thoughts to the test by asking yourself a series of questions about your beliefs about your condition.

4. Where you place your attention is where your energy will go. Do you want to direct your attention inward to address your condition or outward toward the external world?

5. Who do you need to be and show up as in the world to do the work required to reach your goal?

Go Deeper

Awaken the Genius by Dr. Patrick Porter

Thrive in Overdrive by Dr. Patrick Porter

Evolve your Brain by Dr. Joe Dispenza

PART III

Compassion

"*Compassion lies within each of us. What if we first extended sympathy to ourselves for the past and then consciously extended that to others?*"

Dr. Sabrina Crouch

CHAPTER 5

No Success Without Feedback

Notice that I didn't lead with the other F-words like failure or fear. Have you ever asked yourself questions such as: How do I bounce back from adversity? How do I put myself out there to take another chance? What if what I'm doing doesn't work? Better questions to ask instead are: What if I do nothing? What if I succeed beyond my imagination? Is that far more terrifying? When life applies friction, apply energy. Don't get sucked up by the vacuum of regret. If we are asking how or when relief will come or if we will achieve success in healing or changing our condition, we are getting side-tracked. We are not going to concern ourselves with that. It is important to paint the picture as if what you wanted has already been achieved, not only with an affirmation but also with the feeling. In his book *The Art of Mental Training,* D. C. Gonzalez said that in order to be good at whatever you do, you can't be afraid of failing. It all comes down to how your body responds to the emotions of fear. Fear is a heavy and restricting emotion, and combined with our thoughts, we can keep the emotion alive. When people are afraid, they often look for a "sure" thing and lean towards "safety." (I'm raising my hand here.) The only way to accomplish anything is to disempower the fear and grow through the challenge. Dr. Patrick Porter said, "Failure is feedback." Let's use this feedback to pivot and make adjustments.

Think back to times you have taken a chance and tried something outside of your comfort zone or a past medical challenge you have overcome. When I think back to when I was younger, I was more adventurous. I went scuba diving, ziplining, and trained for a 350-mile bike ride from New York to Boston. Now, pushing myself past my limit seems like a chore, but that is exactly what is necessary to stretch the limits of possibility and widen my comfort zone. Yes, that means taking another chance. We are not competing with anyone except our past selves. Why be defined by one moment when we live 31,536,000 seconds per year? Unfortunately, we don't always learn from the experiences of others unless we are ready. We eventually have to learn from our experiences. We can't spare each other the journey. Tim Grover, in his book *Relentless,* said it perfectly; "Failure is what happens when you decide you failed." The real work on this journey requires a new way of thinking. We've been taught to rely on our minds to analyze information. As kids, we all learned to classify and categorize things as right or wrong, good or bad, and black or white. It sounds simple. However, I've come to realize that just because I can't see or think of something with my conscious mind, it doesn't mean that it doesn't exist. Everyone is an expert in what they know, but few acknowledge what they don't know. There might be other possibilities, but they are outside of our awareness.

I appreciate the work of sport psychologist and athletes who train at the professional level. They understand the mental aspect of their game. Someone I admire once said, "Sport transcends life and teaches you a level of perseverance." We can use these strategies that many of us used to use in sports and apply them to our lives now. In the book *On Top of Your Game*, by Carrie Cheadle, she states that athletes understand that they will inevitably encounter challenges along the way; they learn to embrace the entire journey, including the obstacles, challenges, and setbacks. They learn to embrace the errors and losses. The ability to deal with setbacks is what distinguishes a true athlete from their competitors. Although we are not in competition with others on our journey, we can apply this to our situation. What is going to distinguish you from your past self?

The reality is no one can do your work for you. Do you want to reclaim your power? Books, research, and technology can provide you with information, but it is up to you to integrate it and experience it through action in order to see things from a different perspective. In George Mumford's *The Mindful Athlete,* in the chapter Insight, he talks about how you see yourself creates your reality. Your beliefs become thoughts; your thoughts become words; your words become actions, and your actions become habits. You know how hard habits are to break, not only physical habits but also thinking habits. We are not our mistakes, and we are bound to make them along the way. Who is ready to succeed?

"Success is 99% failure."

George Mumford

CHAPTER 6

Changing the Narrative

Your journey to meditation and healing can't be compared to anyone else's. I enjoy hearing testimonials because they fuel me. It doesn't matter if it is only one person's experience or the experience of a few people. What it does for me is reinforce possibility. This was a hard pill to swallow as a psychologist who is trained to critically examine research to determine interventions. No one wants to try something that is not mainstream and research-based, but I had to ask myself, *What is the alternative? Do I sit and wait for my pain to worsen? Do I allow the worst-case scenario to condition me to live in fear?* I was believing in something that I could not yet see. As a patient, after being told that my condition couldn't be cured, I was internally driven to try a different approach. All it takes is one person to have a breakthrough for others to try. I don't know if you saw Breaking Two (2017), about the attempts

> *"Compassion doesn't mean that we don't fight. It just means that we don't hate."*
>
> Sharon Salzberg

46

to break the two hour marathon record but in 2019 Eliud Kipchonge became the first athlete to accomplish something that was previously unheard of. Meditation works for me because I believe it will work; I'm willing to do the work, and I feel I'm benefiting from the work. I trust the science behind these techniques, and although meditation is becoming more mainstream, this is only one part. You have to find a way to embody these techniques and create a new narrative.

Compassion and Forgiveness

Could you forgive if your health depended on it? A John Hopkins Medicine article on wellness discussed the physical burden associated with hurt and disappointment. Studies have found that the act of forgiveness can lower the risk of heart attack, improve cholesterol levels and sleep, and reduce pain, blood pressure, levels of anxiety, depression, and stress. Research points to an increase in health benefits of forgiveness as you age. Yes, I'm going there. As we age and accumulate more layers of experiences that shape us and trigger old trauma, it is more important to work toward forgiveness. Dr. Kristin Neff, a researcher and pioneer in the field of self-compassion, states that self-compassion goes beyond accepting our experience. She adds that self-compassion includes "embracing the experiencer (i.e., ourselves) with warmth and tenderness when our experience is painful."

It is probably easier for most to be kind to others while being judgmental and critical of ourselves. We often hold ourselves to impossible standards. Just as we give others permission to be imperfect, we need to lend that to ourselves. I've often heard it said to treat yourself with the compassion you would give a small child. We may think of compassion as soft, but compassion can be freeing. There are many lessons in forgiveness; one of the most remarkable I've heard was from Immaculée Ilibagiza, a Rwandan genocide survivor. Between April 7 and July 15, 1994, over one million people were killed, including her family and friends. She talked about the process she went through to forgive. Forgiveness doesn't mean what happened was okay. The reason that she needed to forgive was for her. She talked about the price her body paid, and described herself as "aching and paralyzed with anger."

She decided to do what seemed impossible. Through her faith, she was able to find the courage to let go of anger, forgive, and she was left with peace. If she can forgive, anyone can forgive. Immaculée's story gave me some perspective. She overcame the unimaginable.

Kristin Neff, in her 2015 article "The Five Myths of Self-Compassion: What Keeps Us from Being Kinder to Ourselves?" stated that self-criticism and not knowing what self-compassion looks like keep people from practicing it. Common misconceptions about self-compassion included viewing it as a form of self-pity (meaning weakness) and leading to complacency. Others viewed self-compassion as narcissistic or selfish. These are all myths. Somewhere along the way, we adopted the narrative of feeling like we are not good enough, feeling like things "should" go our way, or that other things "shouldn't" happen to us. Compassion, like other qualities, can be contagious. If we can learn compassion for ourselves, it can spread to others. It doesn't have to be attached to religion or spiritual practice. Compassion can be learned and cultivated. On her website, Kristin Neff suggests a few techniques to learn this practice, including writing down your self-talk and asking yourself if you would ever say these words to a friend. Another technique is writing a letter to yourself, taking the perspective of another person, and then reading the letter and receiving those words from yourself. I urge you to look into the comprehensive list of resources and practices to boost self-compassion that are on her website: www.self-compassion.org.

Through my condition, I learned not to be so hard on myself. I was expecting my body to bounce back and be what it was instead of embracing and accepting it. I was expecting it to be the same all day, every day. I wanted it to be "normal." We all know there is no such thing as "perfect" or "normal," but for some reason, we keep buying into the illusion. Compassion, like surrender, does not mean giving up. I no longer have to fight to return to my past self. I can embrace my "now" normal and be grateful. Pain, frustration, and disappointment are all shared emotions. We are not alone in these, and we are all interconnected and interdependent, so there is no need to hide from yourself. If you are reading these words, then you have survived challenges before, and your journey is not over.

Reflections

1. Challenges are inevitable, but we can gain feedback from them, which can help us pivot.

2. Think back to times when you faced other challenges and the lessons that you learned from them.

3. What is one way you can increase your self-compassion? Pick one technique from Kristin Neff's list and journal about the experience.

Go Deeper

Radical Acceptance by Tara Branch

The Art of Forgiveness, Lovingkindness, and Peace
by Jack Kornfield

Techniques to Increase Self-Compassion by Kristin Neff
www.Self-compassion.org

A free online course in Mindfulness-Based Stress Reduction (MBSR) www.palousemindfulness.com

"Forgiveness is giving up the hope that the past could have been any different, it›s accepting the past for what it was, and using this moment and this time to help yourself move forward."

Oprah Winfrey

PART IV

Courage

"*I believe that courage is about finding joy, even in challenging times. It is not about the big triumphs, but the small steps we take each day to honor our spirit and the life energy God gave us. It is all about the journey; you may as well enjoy the ride.*"

Dr. Sabrina Crouch

CHAPTER 7

Surrendering to Rainbows

I remember asking my guide, "Are you sure we can't see the rainbows from the car?" Just the week prior to the trip, my friend suggested a trip to Vinicunca, also known as rainbow mountain. I had never heard of it, but I was willing to go. Everything was going as planned until check-in time at the airport when I discovered that I was going to Peru alone. The funny thing about meditating is that it has helped me to adapt to changing situations. I easily boarded the plane but felt uneasy about the hike. Two weeks before, I was in Bogota, learning more about Dr. Joe's formula. I guess that trip was preparation for this experience. After some back and forth with the guide, I finally surrendered and agreed.

The Hike

It all started in darkness. My first steps were guided by Alex as we followed a beam of light from his flashlight. We were the first two hikers on the path, and the only other people we passed were the park rangers. I posed for a picture lit by a flash, holding two walking sticks. Let me just say that I am not a hiker. I've walked on some trails before but nothing strenuous and never at an elevation of 15,000 feet. I was dealing with not only the terrain but also the air. Quickly, I realized that my body didn't move as fast as I wanted it to at that altitude.

Alex patiently coached me along the way. I knew right away that I had found the right guide. I had no idea that he would be my spiritual guide as well. As we walked, I could feel his connection, reverence, and respect for the land of his birth. He was familiar and comfortable with the unexpected changes in temperature and terrain. He knew what to do at the appropriate time. At times, he remained silent; other times, he talked to me. When he saw my frustration with the steep inclines as I attempted to push forward and then double over to catch my breath, he said, "Walk in a zigzag." He strolled, walking on an angle going one way and then the other. I imitated his movements. At times, when I looked for him, Alex was beside me, or behind me, or in front of me, allowing me space to take it all in.

As dawn appeared, I asked, "Where is the rainbow?" Alex responded, "On the other side." I refocused my attention on my surroundings and noticed a black dog approach us. He was friendly; I remember petting him and thinking fondly how much I enjoyed having a dog growing up. Periodically, the dog would disappear and reappear in front of us. He was so relaxed as he walked effortlessly, and I was jealous. He reminded me of the patience and obedience to the process that I needed to embody. The dog would lie and wait for us to catch up before he continued up the mountain. He led the way to the rainbow.

As the end of the hike neared, I realized I had to stop looking ahead for Alex, the dog, and the rainbow. I thought back to my long-distance cycling days. I reminded myself: *Slow and steady, focusing right in front of me, staying in the present moment.* I could hear Alex's voice in the distance, saying, "You are almost there." His voice sounded closer with each step, but I was not ready to look up until I took that last step and turned to see the rainbow-colored mountain at 16,800 feet. It was cloudy, and the colors weren't as vibrant as what I had seen in pictures, but I wasn't at all disappointed. We were the first two to reach the summit that day. In that moment, I felt free and whole, and I realized I was the brightness on the mountain. What I was seeking was within me all along. I just had to surrender to it.

The Meditation

At the top, Alex said he was going to give me a few minutes to myself to meditate. It was at that moment that I realized I had been meditating all along. The hike was the meditation. Each step of that almost three-hour journey was a walking meditation. I had put the formula into practice without even being conscious of it. The art of settling my body down by regulating my breathing and tuning into my environment was meditation. The feeling of the ground underneath my boots was meditation. The feeling of the wind blowing across my face, the chill in my hands, and the warmth from the sun was meditation. Taking it all in without judgment was meditation. Just acknowledging it was meditation. Unconsciously, I began to trust my body again, and in that time of reflection, my heart opened. It was all an experience of meditation, presence, and acceptance, of surrender. There were all those times I could not use my left hand, and for the entire hike, I did so without any sensations of pain or limitations in movement. Somehow, in the midst of surrender, I found courage that I didn't realize was within me.

As I sat there in awe, I felt gratitude and a love for life, and I realized those were the elevated emotions attached to those intentions that I had set two weeks before in Bogota. I had accomplished three out of four of those intentions. I could hear the words of Dr. Joe in my head. "When you marry an elevated emotion with a clear intention…" What I realized was that the marrying was more of a magnifier, a multiplier. That is how powerful it was for me. Those heavy emotions of fear and anger from the past could not have led me to this place. Although I started out on this journey with the goal to find relief for the pain, and I was able to quiet it, what I received on this unexpected journey was much more than I could have ever imagined. And it was not over, and it is not over.

Reflections

I left the Andes mountains with a renewed appreciation for nature and hiking. Not only was it a humbling experience but also I was able to take my attention off time, connect with nature, and contemplate my place within this world. I was able to embrace the uncertainty of the changing terrain and landscape and embrace each step as different. I achieved a state of flow that many athletes refer to as "being in the zone." Now, the goal is to translate this to other areas of my life and embrace other changing situations. I work at this each and every day and, sometimes, from minute to minute. This physical challenge was just what I needed. In *The Mindful Athlete*, George Mumford stated, "If you continue to push your body in an incremental fashion—ideally practicing intention, visualization, and deliberate practice at the same time—your body will eventually adjust to the new physiological level required of it, thereby increasing your physical capacity."

"You will never live to your greatest potential unless you open your heart."

Paulo Coelho

CHAPTER 8

Rebirth

We are changing beings whether we like it or not. This is how God created us. I feel different, and I'm more aware of my changing and expanding thoughts. I realize that now that I am showing up for myself, I have a raised consciousness as well as a new perception of pain. I used to be upset with it, and wanted to be mad at it, but I realized that I was mad at something that was within me. So, did this mean that I was mad at myself? Perhaps. I find that when I do have pain, I can lean into it. In his article, "Responding to Emotional or Physical Pain," Dave Potter calls this "turning toward." When we turn toward, there is an attitude of curiosity and a willingness to be with and explore and experience pain even if it's uncomfortable. It makes me think and ask myself what is causing my pain to occur. Is it stress or tension or am I doing too much? This is not easy; it takes practice. Occasionally, I can acknowledge the pain and simply return to my breath. Dave calls this "letting go." There are other times when I can be hyper-focused on a task and feel discomfort. Those times, I joke with it and say, "Not now, I'm busy." Maybe, this is a healthier form of what Dave calls "blocking." The point is, I'm now conscious of it. There are a variety of meditations and informal practices that

57

can specifically guide you through learning this process. We have to learn greater tolerance for cognitive dissonance and extend our level of comfort to eventually encompass what was once uncomfortable a few seconds at a time.

I realize that this expansion has not only changed my relationship with pain but also changed my relationships with others. For this, I can't apologize. Some people try to relate to me as the person they remember from the past and connect in ways that no longer work for me. I am firm and unapologetic about my boundaries. It is refreshing when a friend asks, "Can I tell you what I think?" before offering their advice. I smile because it means that people are starting to understand the me that I'm becoming. I love replying, "No." I trust that the answers that are for me will come to me in due time. The answers I truly seek about life are not going to come from outside of me. If I sense that advice is fear-based or about something trivial, I can release it. Remember, people's opinions typically reflect what they would do if they were you. I always feel like I have a choice. Granted, with choices come responsibility. The key is being willing to accept the consequences of your choices as part of your journey. We make choices based on what we know at the time. Looking back, if my choice was not the best, there is nothing I can do about it now. I believe we only have regret if we have not learned a lesson from our circumstances.

"My doctor told me I would never walk again. Mother told me I would. I believed my mother."

Wilma Rudolph

When I reflect on this quote, I realize it sums up much of what I have been talking about: believing in possibility despite a diagnosis or a condition. As a child, Wilma Rudolph wore leg braces, and doctors didn't think she would ever walk again, let alone run. In the 1960s, she went on to become the fastest woman in the world and a world record Olympic champion. She more than overcame her disability; she showed herself and the world her true ability. That's the kind of intention and belief in possibility that we should be planting and nurturing in ourselves and passing on to the next generation. Somehow, I lost sight of that, but on my journey of healing, I rediscovered this power. Now, my pain is infrequent, and I am on a lower dosage of medication. I'm not cured yet (wink), but the pain has quieted tremendously.

On your own journey, you may notice a variety of shifts in your energy and vibration, which mean you are on the right track. It may not look the same for you, but some things that I noticed about myself were:

- Not needing to explain myself or process details with people around me

- Feeling connected to nature and walking around hugging trees

- Feeling grateful even when I was in the midst of what others would see as chaos

- Becoming selective in how I used my energy (nice vs. necessary)

- Choosing freedom over being right when there's a difference of opinion

- Remembering the past and finding the blessing in the lesson

- I'm less likely to take things personally and can make a conscious effort to respond to others with compassion, even if I don't know their story. (This is a hard one. I work at this daily.)

- I'm less attached to outcomes and enjoy the process, no matter how unexpected.

- I am okay with the consequences of my decisions and accept if I knew better, I would have made a different choice.

- I can let go of trying to figure out "how" or "when" something will happen because, in my mind, it is already done.

- I realized we are all connected spirits and feel drawn to a higher purpose.

Change will not always happen when we want it to, but our job is to be ready. Each person can find their own path. We may start out together but veer off in another direction and meet up again at the end. Change is not easy. If it were, everyone would have mastered it. It will require you to not let failure, missteps, or mistakes be viewed or internalized as permanent states. It will take managing fear and using it to pivot in a new direction. It will require a belief in yourself that's not ego-based but based on your true essence. It will take, as Jill Bolte Taylor said in her Ted Talk, *My Stroke of Insight,* "Choosing to step to the right of our left hemisphere." There are new breakthroughs in science every day that stretch the boundaries of our consciousness. Is it possible that you can look at yourself in the mirror and see yourself as more than your body? Our spirit and energy prove that we belong to something greater.

My hope is that this book sparked something within you, and you believe that you can create the life you want that is not defined by a diagnosis or condition. I hope you find possibility in what appears to be an impossible situation. That you can think outside the box of comfort and familiarity, or better yet operate as if there is no box and that your potential is unlimited. Learning to meditate is about changing your state of mind where you can disconnect from the external world and access a new level of consciousness. One of the most profound things I learned on this journey is that each time you get up from a meditation you emerge as a new person. I'm rooting for you and I look forward to seeing who you will emerge as.

Final Words

"You are the artist of your world. Paint it with bright, vivid colors. Be mindful of where your brush strokes. View the bigger picture while paying attention to the tiny details. You reflect the greatness of the universe despite how you may feel at the moment. You are perfectly made. You are a masterpiece."

Wilfredo Torres

Acknowledgments

To my first teachers, my parents, for always encouraging me to believe in possibility. I remember overhearing my father saying to my mother, "You never know, she may be the next Wilma Rudolph." No matter what dreams I had, they were always nearby as I chased them.

Paul C. Brunson, when I joined that Mastermind Group in 2017, I never knew where it would lead me. Thank you for the lessons, and yes, they still resonate with me. This caterpillar has turned into a butterfly.

To my MSU high school sister and executive coach, Angie Correa, for listening to the book idea in March before a single word was written and saying, "Do it."

To my friends Farah Joseph & Adrienne Willis-Connors, for reading and rereading those drafts. Thank you for your love and unwavering support through this process.

To my friends who shared their hopes, dreams, and fears with me as I contemplated sharing mine. Those conversations helped me to know you in a different way and reinforced our spiritual connection.

Wilfredo Torres, I had no idea when I met you that you would bless me with beautiful reflections each morning. They were always right on time. Thank you for letting me share them with the world. Now, I'm ready for you to write that book.

To my Peruvian guide, Alex Carpio, thank you for encouraging me to surrender and introducing me to the beauty and energy of Peru. I carry it with me each day.

To my Egyptian guide and new friend Alaa, thank you for asking me the one question that started me on this journey. I look forward to returning to Egypt one day. I did not forget about Sekhmet. I read she is not only a warrior goddess but also a goddess of healing. How synchronous is that?

To my amazing family and friends near and far whose paths crossed with mine along life's journey. My heart is filled with gratitude.

To my medical team, especially Christine and Sasha, who led me as far as they could and passed me the baton.

Coach Tamara Brown and Chris O'Byrne, you gave me everything I needed and more. There is no coincidence that I was led to you. This journey to becoming an authorpreneur would not have happened without your faith, feedback, and expertise.

To my heart, Mark Pryor, who is right by my side supporting my dreams and vision as I am becoming. I am grateful each day that I can wake up and be my authentic self with you.

#presenceoverpresents

About the Author

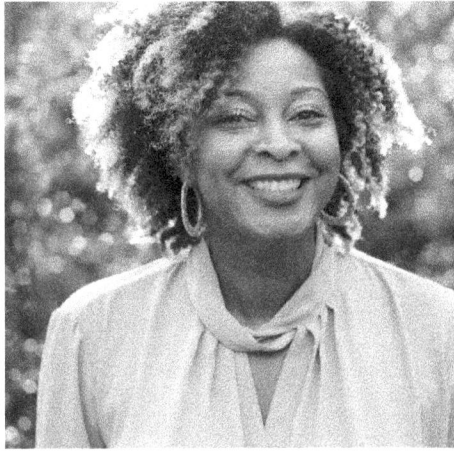

Dr. Sabrina Nichole Crouch is a New York State Licensed Psychologist and Certified Professional Coach. She earned a doctorate in School-Clinical Child Psychology from Yeshiva University, a master's degree from the City College of New York, and a bachelor's from Syracuse University. She is also a diplomate in School Neuropsychology and a Heart Math Practitioner. Sabrina is a lifelong learner and is constantly exploring new endeavors. She is a member of Dr. Joe Dispenza's advanced student community. Outside of her professional accomplishments, she is most proud of her investment in her personal and spiritual development. She has found an opportunity in her challenge of managing chronic pain and can respond to it with curiosity. She has faced the cost of not staying open to change and feels that meditation was the key to transforming her life. In her spare time, she enjoys reading, gardening, hiking, cycling, traveling, and exploring her right-brain creativeness through painting and writing.

www.ingramcontent.com/pod-product-compliance
Lightning Source LLC
Chambersburg PA
CBHW051037030426
42336CB00015B/2928